HOW TO USE MINI HABITS FOR SUSTAINABLE WEIGHT LOSS

DIETING IS UNNECESSARY SUFFERING

FORM NEW LASTING HABITS

Yvonne Findley

HOW TO USE MINI HABITS FOR SUSTAINABLE WEIGHT LOSS

Dieting Is Unnecessary Suffering. Form New Lasting Habits.

Yvonne Findley

Copyright © 2019

Table of Contents

INTRODUCTION 1
CHAPTER 1: DANGERS OF TOO MUCH WEIGHT .. 2
CHAPTER 2: MINDSET AND WEIGHT LOSS 10
   As Per Your Beliefs 10
   Control Emotions To Lose Weight 13
   How Happiness Helps Lose Weight 14
CHAPTER 3: ACCEPTING THE SITUATION 18
   Things You Cannot Change 18
   Things You Can Change 19
CHAPTER 4: LAW OF ATTRACTION AND LOSING WEIGHT 20
   Kind of Changes You Need To Make 21
CHAPTER 5: WATER AND FAT LOSS 23
CHAPTER 6: STAY MOTIVATED TO LOSING WEIGHT 25
   Teach Yourself How To Stay Motivated 25
      Write Down Your Reasons For Wanting To Lose Weight 25
      Get Support From Your Family And Friends 26
      Challenge Yourself 26
      Reward Yourself 26
      Surround Yourself With Positives 27
      Get Help From Your Smartphone 27

Don't Keep Checking The Scales 27
Reduce Sugar Intake 28
CONCLUSION 29

INTRODUCTION

Welcome, ***How To Use Mini Habits For Sustainable Weight Loss***! This book contains proven steps and strategies on how to lose weight and have the body you've always dreamed of by not dieting.

Do you know that you can do anything that you set your mind to do? Do you know that by setting your mind and thoughts to do something, you are merely using the law of attraction? When you set your mind to do something, you align your thoughts to what you want to achieve.

We all want to look the best that we can. However, it's not always possible because we put too many hurdles in the way of our success. Once you learn how to do this, you will wonder why you never discovered its simplicity before. The point is that life throws too many hurdles into our pathway right from the moments of childhood. You may not know it, but your thoughts may be precisely what is getting in the way of really making the most of who you are. Learn through reading this book how you can change all that.

CHAPTER 1: DANGERS OF TOO MUCH WEIGHT

There are so many dangers of overweight that an entire book could be dedicated to just this topic. But as we intend to get a good idea of what we have put at risk, I will list them out here with some explanations as well so that you understand what the concern is and why or how it is dangerous. Here are the adverse health conditions customarily associated with overweight or obesity;

> A. *High Blood Pressure or Hypertension* - Having a high body mass index or extra fat in your body increases your probability of having high blood pressure. Blood pressure is simply the force or pressure that blood exerts on the walls of the arteries as the heart circulates the blood in the body to supply it to every cell to help it meet its oxygen and nutrient requirements. Obesity means that there is extra fat in the body where nutrient and fat requirements must be met and hence to meet the same, more blood must be pumped by the heart to fulfill these additional requirements. More blood in circulation results in higher pressure on the artery walls and hence increased blood pressure.

Now this increased pressure on the arteries or high blood pressure can cause a variety of complications which are listed for your reference below:

1. *Stroke*–High blood pressure over a prolonged period can weaken the blood vessels of the brain, causing them to narrow down and even rupture or leak. Also, sometimes high BP can result in clot formation in arteries that supply blood to the brain, thus cutting off its oxygen supply and leading to a stroke.
2. *Vascular Dementia*–Dementia in simple words is a brain disease which results in problems in thinking, speaking, reasoning, memory, and vision. Narrowing or blockage of the arteries caused by the high blood pressure can result in vascular dementia. It is also sometimes caused by interruption of blood flow to the brain. The cause of both these is high blood pressure which is a result of obesity.
3. *Kidney Failure*–Kidney failure on most occasions caused due to high blood pressure because of the damage it causes to both the large arteries leading to your kidneys and the tiny blood vessels within the kidneys. As a result, the kidneys are unable to filter waste from the blood,

leading to accumulation of large amounts of fluid and waste in the blood which ultimately leads us to either have frequent dialysis or even kidney transplant in the worst case.

4 *Kidney Scarring*–Tiny clusters of blood vessels in the kidneys, called Glomeruli, can sometimes get scarred, leaving them inefficient to filter waste from the blood, which ultimately leads to the same results as above.

5 *Heart Failure*–When the arteries lose their elasticity over time due to plaque buildup or cholesterol or scarring, the heart has to pump harder to get the blood into the arteries. This increased strain on the heart can weaken its muscles over time, and ultimately it may just give up after getting tired of the extra work it must do, which leads to heart failure.

6 *Coronary Artery Disease*–This is one of the most severe problems resulting from untreated high blood pressure caused by plaque buildup in the arteries, which disrupts the blood supply to the heart. High blood pressure means added stress on the arteries, which damages them, making them more susceptible to plaque buildup and narrowing, ultimately leading to coronary artery disease.

7 *Enlarged Left Heart*–High Blood pressure means more work for the heart to supply the blood to all body parts. Due to this extra stress or workload, the heart muscles become stiffer and thicker, which can sometimes make the heart enlarged. This enlarged heart is one of the major causes of heart failure. Since the blood enters the heart from the left side from where it is pumped or supplied to the rest of the body, it is this side that usually works harder and gets enlarged. This condition is also called LVH or Left Ventricular Hypertrophy. People with this condition are four times more probable to suffer a heart attack and twelve times more probable to suffer from a stroke.

B. *Type 2 Diabetes*–The other major result of obesity is diabetes. It is widely observed that overweight or obese people have a high incidence of type 2 diabetes. The reason for it is that being overweight stresses the inside of individual cells, especially the membranous network called endoplasmic reticulum (ER). When the ER has more nutrients to process than it can handle, it sends out an emergency signal to dampen insulin receptors on the cell surface. This causes insulin resistance resulting in consistently high sugar levels which leads to diabetes.

C. *Cancer*-Research has established a strong linkage between some cancers and obesity the usual ones being colon cancer, breast cancer, and cancers of the esophagus, kidneys, and endometrium. Though it is not evident how exactly obesity leads to cancer, it has been statistically found to decrease the cancer risk manifold. According to the World Health Organization, being overweight or obese are the most significant preventable causes of cancer after tobacco. It is guessed that obesity causes cancer by increasing the levels of hormones such as insulin and estrogen.

D. *Sleep Apnea*—It is a disorder in which breathing temporarily stops for 10 seconds or more during sleep. This can rapidly decrease the oxygen levels in the blood and awaken the person during sleep. Obesity is a major cause of sleep apnea because an obese person's airway is often blocked by large tonsils, an enlarged tongue, or soft tissue of the mouth or throat. When asleep the throat and tongue muscles tend to get more relaxed, and that leads to the air passage to be blocked by the soft tissue in the neck (which is nothing but the extra fat that has accumulated due to obesity). A thin person does not face this risk of the air pathway being blocked and hence has much lower chances of sleep apnea.

E. *Nonalcoholic Fatty Liver Disease (NAFLD)*– It is a disease caused by a fat deposit within liver cells when more than 5% to 10% of the liver's weight is fat. It is usually a result of obesity. This can sometimes lead to some very serious liver problems and indirectly to many cardiovascular problems like heart attack and stroke. Sometimes it can lead to inflammation of the liver (called steatohepatitis). And if this hepatitis becomes persistent, it can lead to a more severe condition called fibrosis, in which scar tissue is formed within the liver. And when fibrosis escalates, the structure and function of the liver are severely affected. This condition is called cirrhosis and can lead to liver failure.

F. *Osteoarthritis*–It is the most common form of arthritis which occurs when the protective cartilage on both sides of your bones wears down with time. The most common victims are the joints in hands, hips, neck, lower back, and knees. The simple logic for obesity contributing to this problem is the increased body weight that puts extra pressure on these joints wearing them off even more quickly. It is estimated that being only 10 pounds overweight increases the force on the joint by about 30 to 60 pounds. So even small amounts of weight loss can reduce the pressure on the joints significantly and provide pain relief and prevent further aggravation on joint condition.

G. *Gall Stones*–These are clusters of solid substance that grow in the gall bladder, mostly made of cholesterol. They may occur as one gigantic stone (huge like golf ball) or some minor ones (as little as salt grain). People might not even become aware of their presence in some cases, which means they exhibit no symptoms or cause no pain. Such gallstones are termed silent gallstones. But in many other cases, gallstones cause severe pain in the abdomen, pain under the right shoulder, nausea or vomiting and indigestion after eating high-fat foods.

Since gallstones are cholesterol, there is a direct link between obesity and gallstone as obesity leads to higher cholesterol levels in bile, creating favorable conditions for gallstone formation.

H. *GERD* (Gastroesophageal Reflux Disease)–It is a condition in which the contents of the stomach leak back into the esophagus hence damaging the esophagus lining and causing heartburn and irritation. Studies have shown that GERD is directly linked to BMI (Body Mass Index). During a study, almost 70% of people with a BMI of over 30 had GERD. This dropped down to 5% to 10% for BMI less than

25. That is sufficient to establish a direct correlation between the two.

I. *Gout*—It is a kind of arthritis, resulting from excess uric acid build up in the blood that causes inflammation of the joints. Urate crystals settle in the tissues of joints leading to all sorts of joint problems. It usually affects the big toe but can also affect the heel, ankle, wrist, hand, or elbow. The excess fat in the body leads to uric acid build up as the kidneys cannot keep up with an excess load on them.

J. *Obesity Hypoventilation Syndrome*—It is a breathing disorder affecting some obese people in which weak breathing leads to too much carbon dioxide and too little oxygen in the blood.

CHAPTER 2: MINDSET AND WEIGHT LOSS

The message that you need to carry with you is that you can enhance the positive effect of food and reduce its negative impact on how you think and feel about it. Avoid all foods that you cannot change your feeling about, and eat more of the foods that you can easily have good feelings about. This way, you will never be sorry for what you have eaten, and this is the secret to ensure that whatever you eat has an only positive impact on your body weight.

As Per Your Beliefs

If you believe that your weight loss is going to be a struggle, you are right. If you believe that you are going to achieve the weight that you want to accomplish with great ease, you are right. It happens to you as per your beliefs. This is one lesson that you must learn now, and that will change the way you live life. Yes, it is tough to digest this truth, but the fact is that you will lose weight quickly without much effort if you believe so. But if you think that it's going to be tough, you are going to make it tough indeed to lose weight (just by the power of your beliefs).

You must have sometimes observed that some people do not seem to gain weight even after eating a lot, but some get fat even by breathing in air. So, where do you think the difference is? Wait, if you are thinking their metabolism is fast enough and they burn everything or consume everything they eat quite fast, you are right. It is indeed faster than the ones who tend to gain weight. But what do you think controls our metabolic rate? What decides whether the food we eat will be burned right away or deposited in our body as fat? What is it that decides the fate of the food once it has entered the human body?

Believe me, it is your thinking and feeling about the food you have consumed. It is only and only how you are related to that food. It is only and only how that food makes you feel. It is only the feeling that the particular food invokes. If you are thinking that you are going to get fat with everything you eat, you are ordering your body to do so. You may not put it into words and say it out loud, but if with every piece of food you take in, you crib and murmur, this will add extra pounds to my body and feel bad about the food you eat, it will indeed be deposited as fat.

While eating if you entertain the feeling that it is terrible for you, and it is going to affect you adversely, that is the effect it is going to produce within your body. But this also means that we have been given the power to intervene. We can intervene and impact the effect that the particular food has on our body. Remember that whatever happens in this Universe is as per your expectation of it. You might expect it consciously or subconsciously, but it occurs only as per your expectation. And what you expect is based on your beliefs.

It is therefore advised that whatever you eat expect it to do wonders to your body. Expect it to be digested quickly and accepted by the body. Expect its nutrients to nourish your body. The contents of the food do not matter as much as your expectation of what it is going to do to your body. You might be wondering what you can get away with eating anything bad this way, something high in calories and something believed to be bad for you. Do you need to eat the right things, nutritious diets, and all the good foods? The answer is both a no and a yes.

Would it be possible for you to eat a cake or a pastry or any other food which you are aware is quite high in its calorific value (the number of calories released per unit weight eaten) or any oily food or butter-rich food and still convince yourself that it is suitable for your body? Well if you can do the mental work to convince yourself that such a type of food is good for you, then I invite you to go ahead and eat it with full confidence. It cannot affect you adversely. It will dissolve and disappear in your body like anything. But the fact is that it is tough for us to believe that such food can indeed be beneficial for us and not cause any harm. This is because, over so many years, we have been programmed to believe that certain foods are terrible while others are excellent and still others are midway. Now if we want, we can change this programming. But that will require a lot of mental work, a lot of repetitions, to impress on the subconscious mind the exact opposite of what has been hard-wired into your brain with endless repetitions and reiterations.

It is relatively a lot easier for us to believe the same for a green salad or leafy vegetables or any other raw fresh fruits and vegetables. The conclusion, therefore, is that try to eat what you can feel good about. If it is easy for you to feel good feelings about massive calorie-rich oily food, by all means, eat it. Remember I am talking about what you are feeling inside of you, your most profound belief about it. But if you are like me and like most other people who find it really hard to have such feelings about such heavy food, then the best alternative is go out for the ones for which you can really feel good about, like fresh fruits and vegetables and whatever other food you have learned so far to be excellent or suitable for your health.

Also, even if you happen to eat something that you believe is not that good for you, stop complaining and cribbing about it. The more feeling you create inside of you that you have done something criminal by eating it, the worse the effect the food will have on your body. To summarize it, even if some food has some power to do something terrible to our body, we multiply that power many times by entertaining negative feelings about that food. Instead, if you chose to shower it with lots of love, you will neutralize most of its harmful effects even before it enters your body.

CONTROL EMOTIONS TO LOSE WEIGHT

We have already looked at how stress can affect us negatively causing us to gain weight, and how we can overcome it with the power of gratitude. Well, there are other emotions as well that need to be taken care of. Emotional eating is a huge cause of weight gain. Emotional eating is when you eat for reasons other than hunger; usually your mismanaged or out of control emotions, to feel better in some way. E.g., If you are bored you may munch down a packet of potato chips, if you are sad or feeling low, you tend to prefer sugar-rich foods like ice cream or puddings or pastries because of the instant high it gives you.

These two things make emotional eating more dangerous than eating out of hunger. This is because you are so desperate about what you want to eat that it is difficult to talk yourself out of it. Though you feel the food might be awful for you, but you find it extremely difficult to exercise any self-control and stop yourself short of overeating it. While eating emotionally, you consume a lot more quantity of food and do not stop before you start feeling better, while in eating out of hunger, you will typically stop when your stomach is filled. Therefore, emotional eating is a lot more uncontrolled eating which makes it all the more dangerous. While eating emotionally, we are unable to pick the food that is right for us or restrict ourselves to the right quantity of food.

How Happiness Helps Lose Weight

It is a well-researched fact; that your body functions a lot better, your metabolism is faster, and the body operates more efficiently in every way when you are happy. This is because it is the primary urge of human beings to be satisfied. Most of the things we do are motivated by happiness. The ultimate aim of every goal, every dream is to be happy. The methods, the ideas, or the paths we choose may be different, but the ultimate destination is happiness.

All the organs, tissues, and cells love happiness. This is because when you are happy, you are hormonally very balanced, and this balanced hormone level is the best for the health and growth of your body. Even your cells rejoice and carry out their functions more effectively when you are happy. Hormones are like chemical messengers that have the power to affect our moods and bodily functions. We will also see as to what specific impact each of one has and how it is all related to weight loss. Here is the list:

1. *Serotonin*—This is the primary hormone generally associated with happiness and also sometimes referred to as the 'Happiness Hormone.' It gives one feeling of joy, cures a bad mood, and prevents depression. So, the more serotonin you have, the better your mood and lesser will be mood-related eating. Hence happiness helps control the emotional eating disorder.

2. *Endorphins*—Endorphins are a group of peptide hormones released within the brain and nervous system and influence the way we feel emotionally. Endorphins help fighting stress by increasing our tolerance level for pain and uplifting our mood. We have already seen how stress can lead to weight gain. Combating stress this hormone certainly helps prevent us from picking unnecessary fat. The less stressed we are, the lesser we will eat to

overcome anxiety, and the lesser we eat, the more control we have on our weight.

3. *Dopamine*—Dopamine is a hormone that helps alertness, learning, creativity, concentration, and focus. It is well known that lower dopamine levels leave us craving for food. The body loses weight its dopamine levels drop, which means it craves for food again. Now being happy helps restore the dopamine levels. What it essentially means is that being happy is restoring the dopamine levels in the blood which would have otherwise only been restored by unmindful eating. Therefore, happiness is substituting food in this case as far as hormonal balance is concerned and thus controlling our craving for food. Thus, happiness helps us manage our consumption cravings by regulating dopamine levels.

4. *Phenylethylamine or PEA*-It is a hormone that is a part of many weight loss supplements. It also helps improve mood and mental alertness. It stimulates the release of dopamine that helps in reducing our food cravings. We have already read above that dopamine reduces our food craving, so by increasing dopamine levels, it helps in regulating our food intake indirectly. Since happiness increases PEA, it helps control our food cravings and hence maintain our body weight.

5. *Ghrelin*–It is another stress-busting hormone which helps us relax. The higher the stress, the more is the Ghrelin produced to combat stress. But Ghrelin also increases hunger. Therefore, it increases our appetite, and hence, we tend to eat more while we are stressed. We know that happiness is a great stress buster, so it helps regulate the ghrelin levels by controlling the stress experienced by us. As the ghrelin levels are taken care of, our food cravings or hunger subsides, and that helps in weight loss as we eat lesser as a result.

These are five well-known hormones that are regulated by the amount of happiness, and we have just seen how these relate to our hunger levels, food cravings, and hence weight loss. We have seen at a hormonal level, how happiness helps our weight loss efforts in a big way. Be happy all the time and laugh your way to a healthy lean body. Lay the foundation for happiness, think happy thoughts, and allow the law of attraction to bring you more and happier moments in your life.

CHAPTER 3: ACCEPTING THE SITUATION

THINGS YOU CANNOT CHANGE

You have to learn to accept the things that you cannot change because if you feel that these let you down, you can't think positively and that works against you. You need to be positive at all times. Look into the mirror at your body. You cannot change your hair type, but you can change the style if you wish you. You can't change the length of your legs, so there's not much point in fretting about them. All of the things that you were born with and that cannot change don't even bear thinking about because it is all wasted energy.

In other words, if you want to slim down, you first need to eliminate all of the things that you have so far seen as unfavorable. You can't change them. Forget about having a complex about them because it changes nothing. All it does is make you feel bad about something that is essentially you, and that will never change short of having surgery. Look around you and wake up. People are born with flaws, and they don't all mope about them. Accept those things that you can't change because they are just part of who you are.

You also need to accept why you want to lose weight and keep your aims in mind so that you are positive during the whole process. The problem is that the Law of Attraction won't work all on its own. You have to meet it halfway. When you find that balance that puts you in control of your life, it's incredible. I must say that it took a while to understand the physics of it. I was never that good at sciences at school, but someone put it into diagram format for me, and it was conducive, and I could see how logical it was that if you are not on the same energy wave as the Universe, you can't gain anything at all. We are all one mass of energy, and sometimes negative energy is allowed to take precedence over positive energy. That's when things go wrong.

THINGS YOU CAN CHANGE

You can change your attitude. That's going to be one of the most significant changes that you make. In a future chapter, we will discuss how this helps you and what it does to help the Law of Attraction to work its magic. Once you learn how easy it is, you will wonder why you never did it before. It's not about feeling deprived. You need to work toward something positive and see all the positive sides of being fit and healthy. That's the bit you need to tune into because it's all positive stuff and will keep you in its grasp while you change the shape of your body for the better.

CHAPTER 4: LAW OF ATTRACTION AND LOSING WEIGHT

As per the law of attraction, you merely need to think the things that you crave if you want them to manifest in your life. So, if you are looking to shed the extra pounds, all you need to do is believe that you are already thin and you have a great body that people admire. When you keep murmuring these thoughts to yourself and put away the depressing thoughts of not weighing what you want, you will be able to get the body you have been craving for. Isn't this better than staying hungry all day, opting for crash dieting or spending three hours at the gym? What is the harm in trying it out?

Gone are the days when you needed to give up your favorite foods just to lose a few pounds. Knowing how to vibrate the right kind of energy through changing your thoughts will help you get rid of the extra pounds that you have accumulated. Therefore, you can get a slim shape, which you have been craving for. You can eat your favorite food, skip exercises on days you have no stamina to run, and carve your thoughts in the right direction.

Losing weight is as much a mental thing as a physical one. If you have the confidence of cutting down your extra flab, nothing can stop you from doing it. We'll take a look at some practical strategies to use if you want to enter into the vibrational zone of being fit, which will ultimately make it easy for you to lose weight.

Kind of Changes You Need To Make

When you decide for good that you want a better figure, you change the mindset. Instead of being quite happy to put away the calories, you tend to use a vision board for encouragement and to remind you of what the aim is. This can be something that you don't need to share with anyone else. It's a special thing. Don't add to your unhappiness by trying to measure up to other people's expectations because when you do that in conjunction with weight loss, you tend to set yourself up for failure.

You have to be in this because you want to be in it. Thus, you know common sense ruling about what's acceptable and what's not fair, but the Law of Attraction means that if you already believe yourself to be slim and pretty, the chances are that you will be attracted to foods that actively encourage that. Try your hand at experimentation, but remember that nothing about losing weight in this scenario must be negative. If you find it too hard to resist a temptation, bend to it a little, but not as much as you usually do. A slim and fit lady or man wouldn't eat a whole donut. Therefore, take a bite and keep the rest for another time. That way, you don't have to deprive yourself of anything. You are merely thinking like a thin person and keeping very positive while you do this.

The law of attraction works when you keep a positive mindset. Put the scales away. It's not about you measuring up or being disappointed when you have a bad day. It's about being very happy to be who you are and knowing in your heart of hearts that you can slim down to the weight that you want to be. If you keep showing yourself the positive results of your effort by seeing pictures of what you are inside, rather than what people see from the outside, you really can keep achieving. Think slim. You are slim inside. Now all you need to do is get the outside to catch up. Don't make promises to anyone. This isn't about anyone else at all. It is between you and the picture that you have pinned to your vision board. The point is that you are giving yourself a direction and you are continually positive about it because you know that's really who you are on the inside.

CHAPTER 5: WATER AND FAT LOSS

There has been a ton of research and claims made concerning water and its effect on fat loss. One-minute scientists are claiming that drinking tons of water helps improve fat loss, the next their saying that its effects are minimal and we shouldn't worry about drinking water.

Let's start with the science. Your body, like the earth, is nearly three-fourths water. Most of our major organs are made up of a higher percentage of water than we are. Case in point, the liver, one of the most vital organs we need to survive, is more than ninety percent water. Water is used to move nutrients to the various parts of our body, to oxygenate cells, rid us of toxins, assist digestion, and much more. Without water, we die. It's called dehydration.

Most people live in a state of mild dehydration. We have our coffee in the morning, maybe a little something at lunch and a drink at dinner. That is not enough to stay adequately hydrated, but most of us live such busy lives that we don't even notice we're thirsty half the time. Being dehydrated keeps your body from reaching its peak metabolic state; meaning you aren't burning the highest amount of energy you could be. Without water, your body can't conduct the chemical reactions that use the energy that makes up the sum of your metabolism. So simply by getting away from a typical dehydrated lifestyle will help you lose fat.

However, the benefits don't stop there. Do you know how many calories you take in when you drink water? Zero. It costs you nothing. A bottled soda typically runs anywhere from two hundred and fifty calories to three hundred. For all your calorie counters out there, water is your best friend. It will replace the crap you were already drinking, taking away from excessive calories and nasty fat gaining substances found in the sugary drinks most people suck down regularly. Just because it says "diet" on the side, doesn't mean it's going for. All "diet" implies on soda labels is that it isn't quite as bad as the regular version.

Drinking water also helps you keep your water weight down. Water weight occurs when you retain water because you have a high amount of sodium in your system. The sodium binds to the water as it breaks up. If you have more sodium than water, you end up supersaturated, and the sodium ends up holding onto the water for you. The more water you drink, the more sodium you can break up and the less water you will end up retaining. Drink as much water as you can; you have nothing to lose but excess pounds.

CHAPTER 6: STAY MOTIVATED TO LOSING WEIGHT

When it comes to weight loss, it can be challenging to stay motivated, and weight loss and exercise can become so severe that you could feel like giving up. This is particularly true if you are having a difficult time achieving your goal. It is essential to keep in mind that losing weight is a slow process and it is something that commands complete devotion to achieve your goal, this means that the key to getting rid of your weight and sticking to the healthy eating plan is not about what you eat or the amount of exercise you do but the attitude that you have towards your goal. It is vital to stay motivated and not give up until your goal is achieved. It will happen you can do it.

Teach Yourself How To Stay Motivated

To stay motivated, use the following tips to keep yourself on track:

Write Down Your Reasons For Wanting To Lose Weight

This is particularly important and also the thing that will keep you motivated. Get a piece of paper and write down some of the reason why you want to lose weight and why you need to stick to your healthy eating plan.

There could be several reasons, such as:

To improve your physical status

Reduce the risk to your health

You may want to wear a bikini in front of your friends and feel comfortable about your body. These questions and other similar ones will help you to stay focused and focus on why you started your healthy eating plan in the first place. You should keep this paper somewhere that is easily accessible and read through it every day or every week, and you will be surprised at how much this can help.

GET SUPPORT FROM YOUR FAMILY AND FRIENDS

Working out and staying on your healthy eating plan can become frustrating; however, having friends or family or joining a group of people that share the same goal will be an excellent way to stay on track. The beauty of this is that you will be able to check in with others and discuss the challenges that you are faced with and you can also share ideas on how you can both stay focused and motivated.

CHALLENGE YOURSELF

There are several ways by which you can challenge yourself. You may want to have a competition with your support group as this will provide you all with that little bit of an extra push towards achieving your goal. Set yourself a task; this could be a particular type of exercise or sticking to a specific healthy eating plan. Remember to keep telling yourself that you can do it!

REWARD YOURSELF

It is essential that you reward yourself if you have achieved your objectives or lost a few pounds. You need to find a reward system that works for you. It could be that you take a one or two-day break, or you might buy yourself a new piece of clothing, nail varnish, etc. you get the idea. It is incredible how appreciating yourself will help your motivation to stay healthy.

SURROUND YOURSELF WITH POSITIVES

Act as if you are already the new you. Act as if you are now the person who is at your ideal weight and optimal health. Act as if you are the naturally thin person who always chooses to eat healthy natural foods and quickly says no to processed foods. Act like the person with a higher level of health consciousness by moving your body at least once a day by walking around the block. Arrange your environment to reflect what you are trying to achieve, and this will keep you more focused

GET HELP FROM YOUR SMARTPHONE

There is a multitude of apps that are available for your Smartphone, which can help you to set up a workout routine, get you motivated as well as teaching you new ideas. Download some healthy eating apps that will teach you some of the recipes that you can add to your weekly meal plan and will help you stay on your healthy eating plan.

DON'T KEEP CHECKING THE SCALES

As much as the scales will help you to monitor your progress, frequently using the scales can also undermine your spirit and ultimately kill your motivation. Weighing yourself every day when you are trying to lose weight may provide you with inaccurate results that could be discouraging. Instead, it is better to stick to weighing yourself at the same time once a week.

Reduce Sugar Intake

You need to replace one sugary drink with a tall, glass of water. Our bodies are made up primarily of water, and we need to continuously pump more and more to replace what we lose in sweat. Your body needs optimal amounts of water to function at max capacity and keep you running strong and smooth all day long. Try and find an area where you can make this essential swap that will offer multiple benefits to your health and your life.

Do you drink sugary sodas, flavored coffees, iced mochas, even diet sodas loaded with artificial sugars? If so, these are what we are looking to replace. Don't worry; I am not asking you to go cold turkey and give them up altogether. Start by replacing just one and work your way up from there. By making the switch to water, you will feel full, causing you to eat less. You will feel more hydrated, which has benefits for your mental alertness and skin tone. You will be sheltered from the typical crash that comes along with a burst of sugar, helping you to be more productive throughout the day. Plus, you will save the calories, helping you to lose weight and look and feel better. Now, who doesn't want that?

CONCLUSION

Thanks once again for obtaining this book. It's my firm belief that it will provide you with all the answers to your questions. You need to understand that creating habits is exactly like learning to meditate.

Learning a new habit is precisely the same. You will tumble over obstacles and go back to the old behaviors or habits several times. Why does this happen? What can we do to work past these old behaviors to create new, healthy habits? Initiating and implementing new, healthy habits requires slowing down and becoming self-aware. It also requires a ton of practice, regularity and a heap of self-kindness for those times when we do wander and go back to our old habits! That's bound to happen, so instead of beating yourself up for eating those two pieces of pie and tons of holiday cookies, give yourself a break. Notice what you ate, be compassionate with yourself, and gently return to where you want your focus to be. It is not enough to want to do something differently. It's important to realize that we have been employing other habits of behavior for a very long time. So, be sure to add a truckload of self-awareness, a bottomless pit of self-compassion and a relentless dedication to the regular practice of your new, healthy habits.

I would love to give you some simple steps to make new healthy habits part of your typical routine, but I would be misinforming you if I told you that weight loss is easy. Changing ourselves for the better is one of the most courageous things we can do. So, be kind to yourself. Treat yourself like you would treat someone you love as you attempt the brave act of creating new, healthy habits for yourself!

Hopefully, you will see the underlying value of these simple tips and begin to implement them in your daily life. Enjoy!

Made in the USA
Columbia, SC
31 March 2021